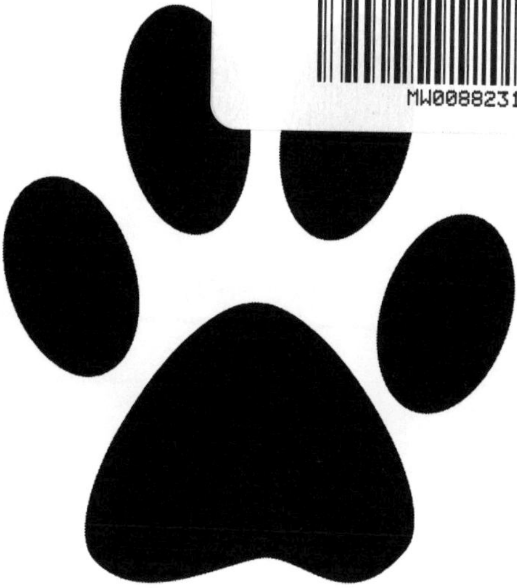

This Journal Belongs To ...

JET VET PUBLISHING

Made in the USA
Columbia, SC
18 December 2019

85312671R00074